Leaky Gut Syndrome Explained: A Syndrome That Is Highly Overlooked But Extremely Dangerous

Disclaimer and Terms of Use: Effort has been made to ensure that the information in this book is accurate and complete, however, the author and the publisher do not warrant the accuracy of the information, text and graphics contained within the book due to the rapidly changing nature of science, research, known and unknown facts and internet. The Author and the publisher do not hold any responsibility for errors, omissions or contrary interpretation of the subject matter herein. This book is presented solely for motivational and informational purposes only.

Table of Contents

Introduction

Leaky gut syndrome is a disease which is caused due to a damaged gut wall or bowel lining. This causes the food particles and toxic wastes to enter the blood stream. Presence of such particles in the blood activates the immune system of the body. This leads to an autoimmune disease which causes severe reactions. This results in several symptoms like migraines, bloating, diarrhea, depression etc.

Leaky Gut Syndrome – Characteristics

- Leaky gut syndrome is a disease which is characterized by a damaged stomach lining. It is a disorder in which intestines are incapable of properly digesting and absorbing food particles.

- The linings of the intestines are directly connected to the blood stream. Any leakage that occurs in the walls of the intestine causes the food particles to flow into the bloodstream.

- In case of a Leaky gut, protein molecules that escape from the bowel linings enter the bloodstream and cause various troubles.

- It is said that along with undigested food toxins, wastes and microbes are also leaked into the blood stream.

- Presence of such unwanted substances in the blood triggers the immune system of the body.

- The function of the immune system is to fight the presence of unwanted substances within the body. In order to fight the foreign bodies the immune system stimulates the release of certain antibodies.

- These antibodies attack various parts of the body and cause several serious symptoms. If left untreated it leads to several autoimmune diseases.

- The immunity system triggers an inflammatory reaction. This results in the production of autoantibody.

- This phenomenon causes several autoimmune responses. This results in severe reactions in the body.

- The theory of Leaky gut is considered as vague by modern medical science. However, the condition of stomach damage in case of patients suffering from auto-immune disease proves the fact that Leaky gut does exist.

- The autoimmune disease caused by Leaky gut results in diseases like Irritable Bowel Syndrome, Crohn's disease, ankylosing spondylitis , multiple sclerosis, dermatitis herpetiformis, arthritis, vasculitis, etc.

- In each of this aforementioned condition improvement in inflammation is accompanied by an equal improvement in autoimmune symptoms.

- Leaky gut syndrome can be symptomatically treated; however, its complete treatment takes time.

- Leaky gut syndrome has yet another name which is known as intestinal permeability. It is believed that on normal basis intestines allow a certain degree of permeability. However, when this permeability exceeds its limits, it results in Leaky gut syndrome.

- Leaky gut syndrome is considered as a serious disease in the field of alternative medicines like homeopathy and Ayurvedic treatments.

- Inflammation of the bowel linings is the major cause that results in intestinal permeability. Hence, treatment is provided to reduce inflammatory reaction.

- Leaky gut syndrome can cause further inflammation and if the condition is left untreated it may lead to severe symptoms like ulcers.

Diagnosis Of Leaky Gut Syndrome

- Although Leaky gut syndrome is a severe disease, it is important to understand that modern science has not recognized this disease as a medical diagnosis. However, it is considered as a proposed condition behind the presence of several disorders. Some of the common disorders are multiple sclerosis and chronic fatigue syndrome.

- National Health Service in UK believes that this disease is unproven and the facts that indicate such a disease are vague in nature.

- Studies have claimed a possible relation between leaky gut syndrome and autism in certain people. This finding has aroused several controversies. However, this matter is a subject of debate.

- An article published in a medical journal in the year 2008, claims that there is a potential relationship between diabetes and Leaky gut syndrome. It was suggested that the findings require more investigation and research.

- Yet another study conducted in the same year suggested a connection between food and nutrient absorption by the intestinal linings and chronic heart disease. Once again more research was recommended to prove the findings.

- The major supporters of Leaky gut syndrome mainly involve nutritionists, dieticians and alternative medicine practitioners.

Symptoms And Signs Of Leaky Gut Syndrome

Since Leaky gut syndrome is often ignored by physicians, its symptoms persist for a longer time. Lack of proper treatment and precautionary measures lead to several symptoms that cause lot of discomfort for the patient. During the initial stages of this disease, the symptoms may be mild. Listed below are some of the symptoms that manifest during the initial stages of Leaky gut syndrome.

- **Bloating:** It is an abnormal sensation in stomach that results in tightness and sometimes pain. It may also cause growling in the stomach. Lack of proper digestion is the major reason behind this symptom. Leaky gut syndrome causes the stomach linings to leak out certain partially digested food particles. Proteins are also leaked out into the blood stream. Owing to partial digestion and lack of absorption, it causes stomach discomfort and bloating.

- **Constipation:** Lack of regular bowel movements causes constipation. Owing to poor digestion the food particles and wastes are not processed by the intestine in an appropriate manner. Lack of enough probiotics also results in constipation. Probiotics are beneficial bacteria that results in proper digestion and absorption of food substances. Since Leaky gut syndrome is an autoimmune disorder the autoantibody produced by the body kills the probiotics and further disrupts the process of digestion. This results in temporary or chronic constipation. A gluten-free diet can help the patient in reducing the intensity of such symptoms. Food items that contain natural probiotics can also resolve this issue.

- **Diarrhea:** Diarrhea is characterized by loose stools, stomach cramps and severe dehydration. In Leaky gut syndrome wastes and toxins are released into the bloodstream. These wastes and toxins are supposed to be excreted by the body. However, their presence in the body may result in infections that result in symptoms like diarrhea. Such situation requires immediate medication. Diarrhea can also lead to dehydration and fatigue. Hence, it is essential to get proper treatment before the situation gets out of hand.

- **Depression:** Depression is a by product of several chronic diseases. Leaky gut syndrome is also a chronic condition that results in severe autoimmune reactions. This causes several symptoms and diseases that result in discomfort and pain. This naturally makes the patient depressed. Leaky gut is also characterized by lack of proper nutrient absorption. Lack of nutrition also causes depression. Besides this, there is a presence of toxic wastes in the bloodstream which causes several chemical reactions in the body. This further causes psychological disturbances and anxiety. And if the disease is not properly identified by the physician the treatment may also take lot of time to bring some affect. Thus the patient tends to be depressed.

- **Intestinal Gas:** Owing to lack of proper digestion, Leaky gut results in the formation of gas. This further hampers the process of digestion and absorption. Intestinal gas causes bloating and flatulence. It can also cause stomach cramps. Medications that aid in digestion can resolve this symptom in 1 or 2 days.

- **Heartburns:** Heartburns are one of the major symptoms of indigestion. It is a burning sensation that spreads across the upper abdominal and heart area. This sensation lasts only for a minute or so. However, they keep on recurring. Acidity is also a major reason behind heartburns. When digestion is hampered stomach produces more acids. Owing to stomach symptoms the patient may reduce the consumption of food. This can also lead to presence of excessive acids in the stomach. Thus there are several reasons behind heartburns. Medications that reduce acidity like antacids are recommended in such a situation. Items like buttermilk and curd can help in reducing heartburns. Drinking lots of water and juices can also help.

- **Gum Diseases:** Gingivitis and gum bleeding are some of the common gum diseases that affect the patients who suffer from Leaky gut syndrome. Presence of toxic wastes in the bloodstream results in several reactions and periodontal diseases are one among them. Proper treatment is required to deal with severe gum diseases and symptoms like bad breath and inflammation of the gums.

In the first stage of Leaky gut syndrome the patient suffers from intestinal swelling. This results in the damage of abdominal coating. This hampers the process of enzyme production. This makes it difficult to digest food. It also affects the process of nutrient absorption. By the time this disease enters its second stage, the symptoms become more severe. Listed below are some of the symptoms that are commonly observed during the second stage of Leaky gut syndrome.

- **Joint Pain:** Pain in the joints can be caused by several changes that occur in our body. Leak gut syndrome is primarily an autoimmune disease. The autoantibody created by the immunity system affects the joints. This causes pain and inflammation of the joints. Treatment consists of anti-inflammatory drugs and pain killers.

- **Migraine:** It is a neurological disorder that causes severe headaches. Lack of proper nutrient absorption effects the secretion of hormones. Autoimmune responses may also effect the secretion of hormones. Hormonal abnormalities are one of the causes that results in migraine headaches. Migraine treatments take time to bring effect. In some cases the medications bring quick relief. However, in certain cases medications hardly bring any changes. In case of Leaky gut syndrome, headaches should be treated with proper pain medications. Sometimes this syndrome also causes regular headaches that resolve quickly.

- **Digestive Problems:** During the second stage of Leaky gut syndrome the digestive problems tend to become more apparent and severe. This may cause chronic bloating, stomach cramps, gas, constipation, acidity and several other symptoms. In such situations, it becomes essential to treat the problems with proper medication. Dietary changes are also recommended. The patient should consume a high-fiber diet that can be easily digested. It is also recommended to have a gluten-free diet. Consumption of gluten-free diet has several benefits. Foods containing probiotics like curd, yogurt and fermented foodstuffs are also beneficial.

- **Dermatitis:** The condition that causes inflammation of the skin is known as dermatitis. It causes itching, redness and burning sensation. This disorder is sometimes referred as eczema. This is a reaction to the autoimmune nature of the Leaky gut syndrome. Treatment with proper anti-inflammatory drugs is essential to resolve this issue.

- **Psoriasis:** Psoriasis results in reddish patches on the skin. It also causes itching. It is a disorder that stems from abnormal immune reaction. Since Leaky gut syndrome results in autoimmune responses there is a chance of developing psoriasis. This condition cannot be fully cured. However, certain immunosuppressant drugs can relieve the symptoms to a certain extent.

- **Chronic Fatigue:** One of the major symptoms of Leaky gut syndrome is chronic fatigue. This results in generalized feeling of weakness and drowsiness. The patient may not feel like undertaking any heavy chores. Lack of proper nutrient absorption is the major reason behind this chronic fatigue. Multiple medications may also induce fatigue and drowsiness. In such situation it is beneficial to drink lots of fluids and consume a nutrient-rich diet. Vitamin supplements and dietary supplements that contain more nutrients are also recommended.

In the third stage, the cells of the intestinal lining begin to breakdown. This results in the formation of gaps. This causes the partially digested food to leak through the gaps. Thus it pollutes the bloodstream and also effects the digestion. The symptoms during this stage are more severe and this takes the form of several chronic issues. Some of the probable results of 3rd stage Leaky gut syndrome are listed below.

- **Ulcerative Colitis:** Ulcerative colitis is a variety of IBD (inflammatory bowel disease.) The word colitis stands for inflammation of the colon. Colon is the last part of the large intestine. The major symptom of this disease is inflammation of the large intestine. In severe cases it also results in ulcers. These ulcers may also lead to open sores that bleed. The major sign of this disease is chronic diarrhea. It also causes bloody stools which indicate the presence of an ulcer. It is important to note that inflammatory bowel disease is quite distinct from that of irritable bowel syndrome. Few of the symptoms of ulcerative colitis are same as Crohn's disease. However, Crohn's disease is more severe as it involves inflammation of the entire gastrointestinal tract. In case of ulcerative colitis only the colon and the large intestine is affected. With proper treatment ulcerative colitis can be cured to a great extent. However Crohn's disease is difficult to be cured.

- **Arthritis:** Arthritis is of different types. In case of Leaky gut syndrome arthritis is a direct result of autoimmune response. This results in inflammation of the joints. The symptoms are joint pain and stiffness. If the condition is left untreated it can exacerbate and cause chronic pain. Proper rest along with immunosuppressant drugs can improve the situation.

- **Systemic Candidiasi:** This is an infectious disease caused by Candida albicans. It causes infection and sepsis. This is also a result of autoimmune response.

- **Onychomycosis:** It is a kind of nail fungus infection that causes discoloration of the nails. Sometimes it may cause pain and inflammation of the skin near the nails.

- **Ringworm:** Ringworm is a fungus that causes skin infections. It is also known as tinea corporis. It causes redness and itching. With proper treatment this fungal infection can be controlled.

- **Celiac Disease:** Celiac disease is a popular autoimmune disorder. It affects the small intestine. Leaky gut syndrome can lead to celiac disease if it is left untreated. It causes stomach pain, diarrhea, constipation and anemia. Chronic fatigue is also a direct result of celiac disease. People affected by this disease are usually undernourished because their small intestine lacks the ability to absorb vitamins, minerals and other nutrients from the food. Celiac disease is related to gluten intolerance. Gluten is a kind of protein which is found in food substances like barley, wheat and rye. Hence, along with medication the patients are supposed to take a gluten-free diet. Consumption of foods that contain probiotics is also beneficial. This can help the patient to get relief from constipation and indigestion. Food supplements that contain probiotics are also beneficial.

- **Skin Disorders:** We have already seen that Leaky gut syndrome can result in fungal and bacterial infections. The autoimmune condition causes several troubles that may manifest in the form of skin disorders. This may include symptoms like swelling, redness, itchiness and inflammation of the skin. Although it may take lot of time to resolve skin disorders, the condition can be controlled with proper medication.

- **Colitis:** Colitis is a symptom of certain stomach ailments like ulcerative colitis. The term colitis basically means inflammation of the colon. Colon is a part of large intestine. The symptoms include stomach pain, bloating, fatigue, cramps, bloody diarrhea, loss of appetite, weight loss, abdominal tenderness and fever. These symptoms may vary in severity depending on the effectiveness of the treatment given. Timely treatment is essential to deal with colitis and its symptoms. It is also essential to have a diet that aids in easy digestion.

- **Multiple Sclerosis:** Multiple sclerosis is an inflammatory disease that affects the nerve cells. The nerve cells are protected by an insulating cover. In case of multiple sclerosis this protective covering is damaged. This primarily affects the nerve cells of the spinal cord and brain. Destruction of the protective layer affects the communication ability of the cells. This leads to several physical as well as mental symptoms. It may also result in more serious neurological problems. A disturbed immune system is considered as the major culprit behind this disease. The sad part is that treatments can bring very little change to this condition. A person effected with multiple sclerosis experiences different types of symptoms like lack of sensitivity, speech problems, visual problems, fatigue, chronic pain, muscle spasms and so on.

- **Crohn's Disease:** Crohn's disease is a kind of IBD (Inflammatory Bowel Disease). It affects the entire gastrointestinal tract; however, the inflammation occurs only in certain areas. Some of the common symptoms of Crohn's disease are stomach pain, vomiting, diarrhea, anemia, weight loss, arthritis, skin rashes and fatigue. Certain patients also experience inflammation of eyes which causes lot of discomfort. In Crohn's disease the immune system fights against the gastrointestinal tract causing severe damage. The disease further weakens the immune system. Although treatments are available to control the symptoms, it is difficult to eradicate the problem in its entirety. Although surgery can offer good relief, in most cases, there is a relapse.

- **Hashimoto's Thyroiditis:** It is an autoimmune disease that leads to inflammation of the thyroid. The immune system of the body fights against the thyroid glands causing severe damage. The condition is difficult to be cured; however, medications can control the disease. Nevertheless, laser treatments have proved effective in restoring the functions of thyroid.

All these aforementioned diseases are a result of severe Leaky gut syndrome. Lack of proper treatment can exhaust the patient's immune system. This leads to different types of autoimmune disorder. Hence it is advisable to take appropriate treatment in an early stage itself. In most cases, physicians are unsuccessful in identifying the disorder of Leaky gut syndrome and they keep on providing symptomatic treatments. This doesn't resolve the situation. Therefore, it is essential to find out the real cause of symptoms and accordingly create a foolproof treatment plan.

Proposed Treatment Methods

- It is proposed that a gluten-free diet and certain nutritional supplements can help in reducing the symptoms of Leaky gut syndrome.

- Dietary supplements, herbal preparations and a controlled diet can help in treating the diseases caused by a leaky gut.

- Homeopathic medicines can help in treating Leaky gut syndrome. There are several drugs in homeopathy that helps in soothing the stomach and intestine linings. It prevents inflammation and makes the intestine strong. Strong homeopathic medicines help in restoring the digestive ability of the gut, and thereby, prevent the progression of this disease.

- Herbal extracts made of slippery elm is effective in treating the symptoms of Leaky gut syndrome. This herb creates a protective coating that sooths the intestines and stomach linings. It also reduces irritation and inflammation. Slippery elm is a popular herb which plays a key role in several ancient medicines.

- Marshmallow root extracts also help in speedy recovery from Leaky gut syndrome. This herb is used in preparing several medicinal preparations that help in treating stomach ailments.

- Echinacea is also an important herb that has been used in traditional medicine for treating a wide range of diseases. It helps in strengthening the immune system of our body and thus reduces the effect of autoimmune responses.

- Peppermint tea is a good solution for treating Leaky gut syndrome. Drinking this tea on a regular basis provides a soothing effect to your stomach and intestines. Peppermint also has strong antiseptic properties which help in preventing several diseases. It also enhances bile flow and thereby aids in easy digestion. Peppermint also helps in curing and preventing infectious diseases.

- **Chamomile Tea:** Chamomile tea is a popular ancient remedy that helps in curing stomach ailments. It helps in curing symptoms like indigestion, gas, cramping, bloating and abdominal pain.

- It is important to adopt some diet changes in order to cure the symptoms of Leaky gut syndrome. Improper dietary habits are one of the major causes of this disease. Hence, you should make some diet changes. You should avoid processed foods that contain too much of additives and preservatives. Junk food that contains lots of fats and calories should be avoided. You should also stop taking carbonated drinks, alcohol and beers.

- Include more fruits and vegetables in your diet. Note that all the food items you take should be well cooked. This aids in digestion and it also reduces the risk of diseases caused by bacteria and microbes.

- Avoid food items that contain gluten. This includes wheat and wheat products like bread. You should also avoid foodstuffs that contain rye, barley and triticale. If you have symptoms of celiac disease then it is best to avoid these food items.

- Include more probiotics in your diet. Probiotics are beneficial bacteria that kill the harmful bacteria in your gut. Probiotics also help in curing indigestion and constipation. You should include probiotic-rich foods in your daily diet. Foodstuffs like yogurt, fermented items and certain fruits contain probiotics in large quantities. You can consult your physician and start taking a probiotic supplement if you feel that you are not getting enough probiotics from food alone.

- You should avoid food items that exacerbate your stomach symptoms. It might take time to identify such foodstuffs but once you feel that your body is not accepting a particular foodstuff you should strictly avoid taking it.

Early identification of Leaky gut syndrome can certainly help you in curing this disease. Proper care and diet control is essential to prevent recurrence of this syndrome. You should keep a close watch on your symptoms in order to understand the nature of this disease.